THIS PLANNER BELONGS TO:

THE GAME PLAN

This battle is yours to win!

Cancer is tough, but you are tougher.

Between the endless doctor appointments, the countless medications, and the general exhaustion of day-to-day life, fighting cancer can sometimes feel like fighting the entire world. Whether you're in the battle yourself or helping a loved one through it, you deserve to have one less thing to worry about. And as you face all these experiences head on, there's one truth underlying all the questions you have right now:

You've. Got. This.

This planner is an organizer, a treatment and medication tracker, a journal, and a weapon in your arsenal as you fight. Most importantly, it is a reminder that you are strong, you are capable, and you are in control of your journey.

Here's how to make the most use of it.

SYMPTOM, HABIT, OR MED	S	M	T	W	T	F	S
Drank water!	X	X	X	X		X	
Headache			X		X	X	
Nauseous	X			X		X	
Yay for keeping dinner down!	X		X		X		

LET'S DO THIS!

Your Treatment Plan & Goals

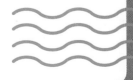

MONTH & YEAR:

SUNDAY	MONDAY	TUESDAY	WEDNESDAY	THURSDAY	FRIDAY	SATURDAY

rise & **SHINE!**
or rise & **SULK.**
or rise & **WEEP!**
or rise & **ROAR!**

BUT RISE.

LIN-MANUEL MIRANDA

What are five small ways to care for yourself,
celebrate, or simply enjoy the month ahead?

THIS WEEK

DON'T FORGET

QUESTIONS TO ASK

TO DO

CHART IT OUT

SYMPTOM, HABIT, OR MEDICINE

	S	M	T	W	T	F	S

MONDAY

TUESDAY

WEDNESDAY

THURSDAY

_____/_____/_____ TO _____/_____/_____

FRIDAY

SATURDAY

SUNDAY

TRIUMPHS OF THE WEEK

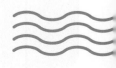

THIS WEEK

DON'T FORGET

QUESTIONS TO ASK

TO DO

CHART IT OUT

SYMPTOM, HABIT, OR MEDICINE

	S	M	T	W	T	F	S
_____							
_____							
_____							
_____							
_____							
_____							
_____							
_____							
_____							
_____							
_____							
_____							

IT'S OK TO NOT BE OK

MONDAY

TUESDAY

WEDNESDAY

THURSDAY

____ / ____ / ____ TO ____ / ____ / ____

FRIDAY

SATURDAY

SUNDAY

/

TRIUMPHS OF THE WEEK

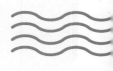

THIS WEEK

DON'T FORGET

QUESTIONS TO ASK

TO DO

CHART IT OUT

SYMPTOM, HABIT, OR MEDICINE

S	M	T	W	T	F	S

GIVE CANCER HELL

MONDAY

TUESDAY

WEDNESDAY

THURSDAY

_____ / _____ / _____ TO _____ / _____ / _____

FRIDAY

SATURDAY

SUNDAY

TRIUMPHS OF THE WEEK

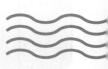

THIS WEEK

DON'T FORGET

QUESTIONS TO ASK

TO DO

CHART IT OUT

SYMPTOM, HABIT, OR MEDICINE

S	M	T	W	T	F	S

GO AT YOUR OWN PACE

MONDAY

TUESDAY

WEDNESDAY

THURSDAY

_____ / _____ / _____ TO _____ / _____ / _____

FRIDAY

SATURDAY

SUNDAY

TRIUMPHS OF THE WEEK

SUNDAY	MONDAY	TUESDAY	WEDNESDAY	THURSDAY	FRIDAY	SATURDAY

If your
COMPASSION
does not include
YOURSELF,
it is incomplete.

JACK KORNFIELD

What are five small ways to care for yourself,
celebrate, or simply enjoy the month ahead?

THIS WEEK

DON'T FORGET

QUESTIONS TO ASK

TO DO

CHART IT OUT

SYMPTOM, HABIT, OR MEDICINE

	S	M	T	W	T	F	S
_____							
_____							
_____							
_____							
_____							
_____							
_____							
_____							
_____							
_____							
_____							
_____							

YOU'RE A FORCE TO RECKON WITH

MONDAY

TUESDAY

WEDNESDAY

THURSDAY

_____ / _____ / _____ TO _____ / _____ / _____

FRIDAY

SATURDAY

SUNDAY

TRIUMPHS OF THE WEEK

THIS WEEK

DON'T FORGET

QUESTIONS TO ASK

TO DO

CHART IT OUT

SYMPTOM, HABIT, OR MEDICINE

	S	M	T	W	T	F	S

EVERY DAY IS A FRESH START

MONDAY

TUESDAY

WEDNESDAY

THURSDAY

_____ / _____ / _____ TO _____ / _____ / _____

FRIDAY

SATURDAY

SUNDAY

TRIUMPHS OF THE WEEK

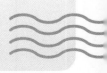

THIS WEEK

DON'T FORGET

QUESTIONS TO ASK

TO DO

CHART IT OUT

SYMPTOM, HABIT, OR MEDICINE

	S	M	T	W	T	F	S
_____							
_____							
_____							
_____							
_____							
_____							
_____							
_____							
_____							
_____							
_____							
_____							

NEVER A VICTIM

MONDAY

TUESDAY

WEDNESDAY

THURSDAY

_____ / _____ / _____ TO _____ / _____ / _____

FRIDAY

SATURDAY

SUNDAY

TRIUMPHS OF THE WEEK

THIS WEEK

DON'T FORGET

QUESTIONS TO ASK

TO DO

CHART IT OUT

SYMPTOM, HABIT, OR MEDICINE	S	M	T	W	T	F	S
_____							
_____							
_____							
_____							
_____							
_____							
_____							
_____							
_____							
_____							
_____							
_____							

ONE DAY AT A TIME

MONDAY

TUESDAY

WEDNESDAY

THURSDAY

_____ / _____ / _____ TO _____ / _____ / _____

FRIDAY

SATURDAY

SUNDAY

TRIUMPHS OF THE WEEK

MONTH & YEAR:

SUNDAY	MONDAY	TUESDAY	WEDNESDAY	THURSDAY	FRIDAY	SATURDAY

If you get tired,
learn to **REST,**
not to **QUIT.**

BANKSY

What are five small ways to care for yourself,
celebrate, or simply enjoy the month ahead?

THIS WEEK

DON'T FORGET

QUESTIONS TO ASK

TO DO

CHART IT OUT

SYMPTOM, HABIT, OR MEDICINE

	S	M	T	W	T	F	S

START WHERE YOU ARE

MONDAY

TUESDAY

WEDNESDAY

THURSDAY

_____ / _____ / _____ TO _____ / _____ / _____

FRIDAY

SATURDAY

SUNDAY

TRIUMPHS OF THE WEEK

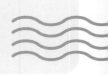

THIS WEEK

DON'T FORGET

QUESTIONS TO ASK

TO DO

CHART IT OUT

SYMPTOM, HABIT, OR MEDICINE

	S	M	T	W	T	F	S
_____							
_____							
_____							
_____							
_____							
_____							
_____							
_____							
_____							
_____							
_____							
_____							

CRUSH IT

MONDAY

TUESDAY

WEDNESDAY

THURSDAY

_____ / _____ / _____ TO _____ / _____ / _____

FRIDAY

SATURDAY

SUNDAY

TRIUMPHS OF THE WEEK

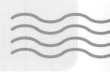

THIS WEEK

DON'T FORGET

QUESTIONS TO ASK

TO DO

CHART IT OUT

SYMPTOM, HABIT, OR MEDICINE

S	M	T	W	T	F	S

BE KIND TO YOURSELF

MONDAY

TUESDAY

WEDNESDAY

THURSDAY

_____ / _____ / _____ TO _____ / _____ / _____

FRIDAY

SATURDAY

SUNDAY

TRIUMPHS OF THE WEEK

THIS WEEK

DON'T FORGET

QUESTIONS TO ASK

TO DO

CHART IT OUT

SYMPTOM, HABIT, OR MEDICINE

	S	M	T	W	T	F	S
_____							
_____							
_____							
_____							
_____							
_____							
_____							
_____							
_____							
_____							
_____							
_____							

YOU'VE GOT THIS

MONDAY

TUESDAY

WEDNESDAY

THURSDAY

_____ / _____ / _____ TO _____ / _____ / _____

FRIDAY

SATURDAY

SUNDAY

TRIUMPHS OF THE WEEK

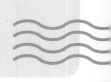

THIS WEEK

DON'T FORGET

QUESTIONS TO ASK

TO DO

CHART IT OUT

SYMPTOM, HABIT, OR MEDICINE

	S	M	T	W	T	F	S

_____

_____

_____

_____

_____

_____

_____

_____

_____

_____

_____

NEVER GIVE UP

MONDAY

TUESDAY

WEDNESDAY

THURSDAY

_____ / _____ / _____ TO _____ / _____ / _____

○ FRIDAY

○ SATURDAY

○ SUNDAY

TRIUMPHS OF THE WEEK

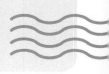

SUNDAY	MONDAY	TUESDAY	WEDNESDAY	THURSDAY	FRIDAY	SATURDAY

Expect trouble as an inevitable
part of life, and when it comes,

HOLD YOUR HEAD HIGH,

look it squarely in the eye, and
say, "I will be bigger than you.

YOU CANNOT DEFEAT ME."

ANN LANDERS

What are five small ways to care for yourself,
celebrate, or simply enjoy the month ahead?

THIS WEEK

DON'T FORGET

QUESTIONS TO ASK

TO DO

CHART IT OUT

SYMPTOM, HABIT, OR MEDICINE

S	M	T	W	T	F	S

FOCUS ON WHAT HELPS YOU

MONDAY

TUESDAY

WEDNESDAY

THURSDAY

_____ / _____ / _____ TO _____ / _____ / _____

FRIDAY

SATURDAY

SUNDAY

TRIUMPHS OF THE WEEK

THIS WEEK

DON'T FORGET

QUESTIONS TO ASK

TO DO

CHART IT OUT

SYMPTOM, HABIT, OR MEDICINE

	S	M	T	W	T	F	S

BELIEVE IN YOURSELF

MONDAY

TUESDAY

WEDNESDAY

THURSDAY

_____ / _____ / _____ TO _____ / _____ / _____

◯ FRIDAY

_____

◯ SATURDAY

_____

◯ SUNDAY

TRIUMPHS OF THE WEEK

THIS WEEK

DON'T FORGET

QUESTIONS TO ASK

TO DO

CHART IT OUT

SYMPTOM, HABIT, OR MEDICINE

S	M	T	W	T	F	S

_____

_____

_____

_____

_____

_____

_____

_____

_____

_____

_____

YOU ARE LOVED

MONDAY

TUESDAY

WEDNESDAY

THURSDAY

_____ / _____ / _____ TO _____ / _____ / _____

FRIDAY

SATURDAY

SUNDAY

TRIUMPHS OF THE WEEK

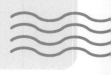

THIS WEEK

DON'T FORGET

QUESTIONS TO ASK

TO DO

CHART IT OUT

SYMPTOM, HABIT, OR MEDICINE

	S	M	T	W	T	F	S

FIGHT LIKE A BOSS

MONDAY

TUESDAY

WEDNESDAY

THURSDAY

_____ / _____ / _____ TO _____ / _____ / _____

FRIDAY

SATURDAY

SUNDAY

TRIUMPHS OF THE WEEK

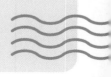

MONTH & YEAR:

SUNDAY	MONDAY	TUESDAY	WEDNESDAY	THURSDAY	FRIDAY	SATURDAY

There is no normal life that is free of pain. It's the very wrestling with our problems that can be the **IMPETUS** for our **GROWTH.**

FRED ROGERS

What are five small ways to care for yourself, celebrate, or simply enjoy the month ahead?

THIS WEEK

DON'T FORGET

QUESTIONS TO ASK

TO DO

CHART IT OUT

SYMPTOM, HABIT, OR MEDICINE

	S	M	T	W	T	F	S

MAKE IT HAPPEN

MONDAY

TUESDAY

WEDNESDAY

THURSDAY

_____ / _____ / _____ TO _____ / _____ / _____

FRIDAY

SATURDAY

SUNDAY

TRIUMPHS OF THE WEEK

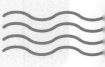

THIS WEEK

DON'T FORGET

QUESTIONS TO ASK

TO DO

CHART IT OUT

SYMPTOM, HABIT, OR MEDICINE

	S	M	T	W	T	F	S

JUST BREATHE

MONDAY

TUESDAY

WEDNESDAY

THURSDAY

_____ / _____ / _____ TO _____ / _____ / _____

FRIDAY

SATURDAY

SUNDAY

TRIUMPHS OF THE WEEK

THIS WEEK

DON'T FORGET

QUESTIONS TO ASK

TO DO

CHART IT OUT

SYMPTOM, HABIT, OR MEDICINE

	S	M	T	W	T	F	S

	S	M	T	W	T	F	S

| | | | | | | | |
| | | | | | | | |

| | | | | | | | |
| | | | | | | | |

| | | | | | | | |
| | | | | | | | |

| | | | | | | | |
| | | | | | | | |

| | | | | | | | |
| | | | | | | | |

| | | | | | | | |
| | | | | | | | |

| | | | | | | | |
| | | | | | | | |

| | | | | | | | |
| | | | | | | | |

| | | | | | | | |
| | | | | | | | |

| | | | | | | | |
| | | | | | | | |

YOU WRITE YOUR OWN STORY

MONDAY

TUESDAY

WEDNESDAY

THURSDAY

_____ / _____ / _____ TO _____ / _____ / _____

FRIDAY

SATURDAY

SUNDAY

TRIUMPHS OF THE WEEK

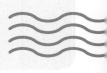

THIS WEEK

DON'T FORGET

QUESTIONS TO ASK

TO DO

CHART IT OUT

SYMPTOM, HABIT, OR MEDICINE	S	M	T	W	T	F	S
_____							
_____							
_____							
_____							
_____							
_____							
_____							
_____							
_____							
_____							
_____							
_____							

HANG IN THERE

MONDAY

TUESDAY

WEDNESDAY

THURSDAY

_____ / _____ / _____ TO _____ / _____ / _____

FRIDAY

SATURDAY

SUNDAY

TRIUMPHS OF THE WEEK

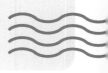

THIS WEEK

DON'T FORGET

QUESTIONS TO ASK

TO DO

CHART IT OUT

SYMPTOM, HABIT, OR MEDICINE

	S	M	T	W	T	F	S

_____

	S	M	T	W	T	F	S

_____

_____

_____

_____

_____

_____

_____

_____

_____

_____

_____

FOCUS ON BEATING THIS

MONDAY

TUESDAY

WEDNESDAY

THURSDAY

_____ / _____ / _____ TO _____ / _____ / _____

FRIDAY

SATURDAY

SUNDAY

TRIUMPHS OF THE WEEK

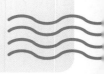

MONTH & YEAR:

SUNDAY	MONDAY	TUESDAY	WEDNESDAY	THURSDAY	FRIDAY	SATURDAY

IN THE DEPTHS OF
WINTER,
I finally learned that within me there lay
AN INVINCIBLE
SUMMER

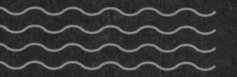

ALBERT CAMUS

What are five small ways to care for yourself,
celebrate, or simply enjoy the month ahead?

THIS WEEK

DON'T FORGET

QUESTIONS TO ASK

TO DO

CHART IT OUT

SYMPTOM, HABIT, OR MEDICINE

	S	M	T	W	T	F	S

HOPE IS NOT CANCELED

MONDAY

TUESDAY

WEDNESDAY

THURSDAY

_____ / _____ / _____ TO _____ / _____ / _____

FRIDAY

SATURDAY

SUNDAY

TRIUMPHS OF THE WEEK

THIS WEEK

DON'T FORGET

QUESTIONS TO ASK

TO DO

CHART IT OUT

SYMPTOM, HABIT, OR MEDICINE

	S	M	T	W	T	F	S

RIDE THE WAVE

MONDAY

TUESDAY

WEDNESDAY

THURSDAY

_____ / _____ / _____ TO _____ / _____ / _____

FRIDAY

SATURDAY

SUNDAY

TRIUMPHS OF THE WEEK

THIS WEEK

DON'T FORGET

QUESTIONS TO ASK

TO DO

CHART IT OUT

SYMPTOM, HABIT, OR MEDICINE

	S	M	T	W	T	F	S

EVERY DAY IS A VICTORY

MONDAY

TUESDAY

WEDNESDAY

THURSDAY

_____ / _____ / _____ TO _____ / _____ / _____

FRIDAY

SATURDAY

SUNDAY

TRIUMPHS OF THE WEEK

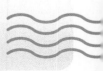

THIS WEEK

DON'T FORGET

QUESTIONS TO ASK

TO DO

CHART IT OUT

SYMPTOM, HABIT, OR MEDICINE

	S	M	T	W	T	F	S

FIGHT CANCER

MONDAY

TUESDAY

WEDNESDAY

THURSDAY

_____ / _____ / _____ TO _____ / _____ / _____

FRIDAY

SATURDAY

SUNDAY

TRIUMPHS OF THE WEEK

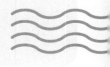

SUNDAY	MONDAY	TUESDAY	WEDNESDAY	THURSDAY	FRIDAY	SATURDAY

You have within you, right now,

EVERYTHING

you need to deal with

WHATEVER

the world can throw at you.

BRIAN TRACY

What are five small ways to care for yourself,
celebrate, or simply enjoy the month ahead?

THIS WEEK

DON'T FORGET

QUESTIONS TO ASK

TO DO

CHART IT OUT

SYMPTOM, HABIT, OR MEDICINE

	S	M	T	W	T	F	S

DON'T YOU DARE QUIT

MONDAY

TUESDAY

WEDNESDAY

THURSDAY

_____ / _____ / _____ TO _____ / _____ / _____

FRIDAY

SATURDAY

SUNDAY

TRIUMPHS OF THE WEEK

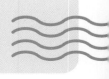

THIS WEEK

DON'T FORGET

QUESTIONS TO ASK

TO DO

CHART IT OUT

SYMPTOM, HABIT, OR MEDICINE

S	M	T	W	T	F	S

IT'S OK TO BE MAD

MONDAY

TUESDAY

WEDNESDAY

THURSDAY

_____ / _____ / _____ TO _____ / _____ / _____

FRIDAY

SATURDAY

SUNDAY

TRIUMPHS OF THE WEEK

THIS WEEK

DON'T FORGET

QUESTIONS TO ASK

TO DO

CHART IT OUT

SYMPTOM, HABIT, OR MEDICINE

	S	M	T	W	T	F	S

	S	M	T	W	T	F	S

BE PATIENT AND TAKE CARE

MONDAY

TUESDAY

WEDNESDAY

THURSDAY

_____/_____/_____ TO _____/_____/_____

○ FRIDAY

○ SATURDAY

○ SUNDAY

TRIUMPHS OF THE WEEK

THIS WEEK

DON'T FORGET

QUESTIONS TO ASK

TO DO

CHART IT OUT

SYMPTOM, HABIT, OR MEDICINE

	S	M	T	W	T	F	S

CANCER CAN'T TOUCH THIS

MONDAY

TUESDAY

WEDNESDAY

THURSDAY

_____ / _____ / _____ TO _____ / _____ / _____

○ FRIDAY

○ SATURDAY

○ SUNDAY

TRIUMPHS OF THE WEEK

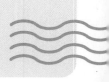

THIS WEEK

DON'T FORGET

QUESTIONS TO ASK

TO DO

CHART IT OUT

SYMPTOM, HABIT, OR MEDICINE

	S	M	T	W	T	F	S

DON'T PANIC

MONDAY

TUESDAY

WEDNESDAY

THURSDAY

_____ / _____ / _____ TO _____ / _____ / _____

○ FRIDAY

○ SATURDAY

○ SUNDAY

TRIUMPHS OF THE WEEK

MONTH & YEAR:

SUNDAY	MONDAY	TUESDAY	WEDNESDAY	THURSDAY	FRIDAY	SATURDAY

None of us know what we are
CAPABLE OF
until we are
TESTED.

ELIZABETH BLACKWELL

What are five small ways to care for yourself, celebrate, or simply enjoy the month ahead?

THIS WEEK

DON'T FORGET

QUESTIONS TO ASK

TO DO

CHART IT OUT

SYMPTOM, HABIT, OR MEDICINE

	S	M	T	W	T	F	S
_____							
_____							
_____							
_____							
_____							
_____							
_____							
_____							
_____							
_____							
_____							
_____							

KEEP CALM AND FIGHT ON

MONDAY

TUESDAY

WEDNESDAY

THURSDAY

_____ / _____ / _____ TO _____ / _____ / _____

FRIDAY

SATURDAY

SUNDAY

TRIUMPHS OF THE WEEK

THIS WEEK

DON'T FORGET

QUESTIONS TO ASK

TO DO

CHART IT OUT

SYMPTOM, HABIT, OR MEDICINE

S	M	T	W	T	F	S

TODAY IS YOURS TO WIN

MONDAY

TUESDAY

WEDNESDAY

THURSDAY

_____ / _____ / _____ TO _____ / _____ / _____

FRIDAY

SATURDAY

SUNDAY

TRIUMPHS OF THE WEEK

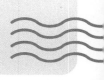

THIS WEEK

DON'T FORGET

QUESTIONS TO ASK

TO DO

CHART IT OUT

SYMPTOM, HABIT, OR MEDICINE

	S	M	T	W	T	F	S

HOPE IS BRAVE

MONDAY

TUESDAY

WEDNESDAY

THURSDAY

_____ / _____ / _____ TO _____ / _____ / _____

FRIDAY

SATURDAY

SUNDAY

TRIUMPHS OF THE WEEK

THIS WEEK

DON'T FORGET

QUESTIONS TO ASK

TO DO

CHART IT OUT

SYMPTOM, HABIT, OR MEDICINE

	S	M	T	W	T	F	S

PROGRESS OVER PERFECTION

MONDAY

TUESDAY

WEDNESDAY

THURSDAY

_____ / _____ / _____ TO _____ / _____ / _____

FRIDAY

SATURDAY

SUNDAY

TRIUMPHS OF THE WEEK

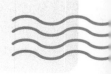

SUNDAY	MONDAY	TUESDAY	WEDNESDAY	THURSDAY	FRIDAY	SATURDAY

What lies **BEHIND US**

and what lies **BEFORE US**

are tiny matters
compared to what lies **WITHIN US.**

HENRY STANLEY HASKINS

What are five small ways to care for yourself,
celebrate, or simply enjoy the month ahead?

THIS WEEK

DON'T FORGET

QUESTIONS TO ASK

TO DO

CHART IT OUT

SYMPTOM, HABIT, OR MEDICINE

S	M	T	W	T	F	S

WARRIOR, NOT A WORRIER

MONDAY

TUESDAY

WEDNESDAY

THURSDAY

_____ / _____ / _____ TO _____ / _____ / _____

FRIDAY

SATURDAY

SUNDAY

TRIUMPHS OF THE WEEK

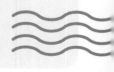

THIS WEEK

DON'T FORGET

QUESTIONS TO ASK

TO DO

CHART IT OUT

SYMPTOM, HABIT, OR MEDICINE

	S	M	T	W	T	F	S
_____							
_____							
_____							
_____							
_____							
_____							
_____							
_____							
_____							
_____							
_____							
_____							

FOCUS ON GOOD THOUGHTS

MONDAY

TUESDAY

WEDNESDAY

THURSDAY

_____ / _____ / _____ TO _____ / _____ / _____

FRIDAY

SATURDAY

SUNDAY

TRIUMPHS OF THE WEEK

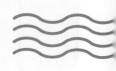

THIS WEEK

DON'T FORGET

QUESTIONS TO ASK

TO DO

CHART IT OUT

SYMPTOM, HABIT, OR MEDICINE

S	M	T	W	T	F	S

FORTUNE FAVORS THE BRAVE

MONDAY

TUESDAY

WEDNESDAY

THURSDAY

_____ / _____ / _____ TO _____ / _____ / _____

FRIDAY

SATURDAY

SUNDAY

TRIUMPHS OF THE WEEK

THIS WEEK

DON'T FORGET

QUESTIONS TO ASK

TO DO

CHART IT OUT

SYMPTOM, HABIT, OR MEDICINE

S	M	T	W	T	F	S

_____

_____

_____

_____

_____

_____

_____

_____

_____

_____

_____

_____

ENJOY THE MOMENT

MONDAY

TUESDAY

WEDNESDAY

THURSDAY

_____ / _____ / _____ TO _____ / _____ / _____

FRIDAY

SATURDAY

SUNDAY

TRIUMPHS OF THE WEEK

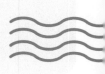

THIS WEEK

DON'T FORGET

QUESTIONS TO ASK

TO DO

CHART IT OUT

SYMPTOM, HABIT, OR MEDICINE

S	M	T	W	T	F	S

KEEP GOING

MONDAY

TUESDAY

WEDNESDAY

THURSDAY

_____ / _____ / _____ TO _____ / _____ / _____

FRIDAY

SATURDAY

SUNDAY

TRIUMPHS OF THE WEEK

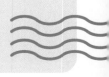

MONTH & YEAR:

SUNDAY	MONDAY	TUESDAY	WEDNESDAY	THURSDAY	FRIDAY	SATURDAY

If you fell down
YESTERDAY,
stand up
TODAY.

H. G. WELLS

What are five small ways to care for yourself, celebrate, or simply enjoy the month ahead?

THIS WEEK

DON'T FORGET

QUESTIONS TO ASK

TO DO

CHART IT OUT

SYMPTOM, HABIT, OR MEDICINE

	S	M	T	W	T	F	S
_____							
_____							
_____							
_____							
_____							
_____							
_____							
_____							
_____							
_____							
_____							
_____							

CANCER SUCKS

MONDAY

TUESDAY

WEDNESDAY

THURSDAY

_____ / _____ / _____ TO _____ / _____ / _____

FRIDAY

SATURDAY

SUNDAY

TRIUMPHS OF THE WEEK

THIS WEEK

DON'T FORGET

QUESTIONS TO ASK

TO DO

CHART IT OUT

SYMPTOM, HABIT, OR MEDICINE

	S	M	T	W	T	F	S
_____							
_____							
_____							
_____							
_____							
_____							
_____							
_____							
_____							
_____							
_____							
_____							

DON'T STOP BELIEVING

MONDAY

TUESDAY

WEDNESDAY

THURSDAY

_____ / _____ / _____ TO _____ / _____ / _____

FRIDAY

SATURDAY

SUNDAY

TRIUMPHS OF THE WEEK

THIS WEEK

DON'T FORGET

QUESTIONS TO ASK

TO DO

CHART IT OUT

SYMPTOM, HABIT, OR MEDICINE   S   M   T   W   T   F   S

_____

_____

_____

_____

_____

_____

_____

_____

_____

_____

_____

_____

YOU ARE STRONGER THAN THIS

MONDAY

TUESDAY

WEDNESDAY

THURSDAY

_____ / _____ / _____ TO _____ / _____ / _____

FRIDAY

SATURDAY

SUNDAY

TRIUMPHS OF THE WEEK

THIS WEEK

DON'T FORGET

QUESTIONS TO ASK

TO DO

CHART IT OUT

SYMPTOM, HABIT, OR MEDICINE

S	M	T	W	T	F	S

POSITIVITY IS A SUPERPOWER

MONDAY

TUESDAY

WEDNESDAY

THURSDAY

_____ / _____ / _____ TO _____ / _____ / _____

FRIDAY

SATURDAY

SUNDAY

TRIUMPHS OF THE WEEK

SUNDAY	MONDAY	TUESDAY	WEDNESDAY	THURSDAY	FRIDAY	SATURDAY

It is only in our

DARKEST HOURS

that we may discover the true strength of the

BRILLIANT LIGHT

within ourselves that can never, ever be dimmed.

DOE ZANTAMATA

What are five small ways to care for yourself,
celebrate, or simply enjoy the month ahead?

THIS WEEK

DON'T FORGET

QUESTIONS TO ASK

TO DO

CHART IT OUT

SYMPTOM, HABIT, OR MEDICINE

	S	M	T	W	T	F	S

IT'S OK TO REST

MONDAY

TUESDAY

WEDNESDAY

THURSDAY

_____ / _____ / _____ TO _____ / _____ / _____

FRIDAY

SATURDAY

SUNDAY

TRIUMPHS OF THE WEEK

THIS WEEK

DON'T FORGET

QUESTIONS TO ASK

TO DO

CHART IT OUT

SYMPTOM, HABIT, OR MEDICINE

	S	M	T	W	T	F	S
_____							
_____							
_____							
_____							
_____							
_____							
_____							
_____							
_____							
_____							
_____							
_____							

SURRENDER? NO WAY

MONDAY

TUESDAY

WEDNESDAY

THURSDAY

____ / ____ / ____ TO ____ / ____ / ____

FRIDAY

SATURDAY

SUNDAY

TRIUMPHS OF THE WEEK

THIS WEEK

DON'T FORGET

QUESTIONS TO ASK

TO DO

SYMPTOM, HABIT, OR MEDICINE

S	M	T	W	T	F	S

NO ONE FIGHTS ALONE

MONDAY

TUESDAY

WEDNESDAY

THURSDAY

_____ / _____ / _____ TO _____ / _____ / _____

FRIDAY

SATURDAY

SUNDAY

TRIUMPHS OF THE WEEK

THIS WEEK

DON'T FORGET

QUESTIONS TO ASK

TO DO

CHART IT OUT

SYMPTOM, HABIT, OR MEDICINE

	S	M	T	W	T	F	S

YOU CAN AND YOU WILL

MONDAY

TUESDAY

WEDNESDAY

THURSDAY

_____ / _____ / _____ TO _____ / _____ / _____

○ FRIDAY

○ SATURDAY

○ SUNDAY

TRIUMPHS OF THE WEEK

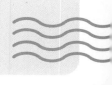

MONTH & YEAR:

SUNDAY	MONDAY	TUESDAY	WEDNESDAY	THURSDAY	FRIDAY	SATURDAY

The way you
TELL YOUR STORY
to yourself matters.

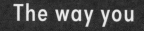

AMY CUDDY

What are five small ways to care for yourself,
celebrate, or simply enjoy the month ahead?

THIS WEEK

DON'T FORGET

QUESTIONS TO ASK

TO DO

CHART IT OUT

SYMPTOM, HABIT, OR MEDICINE

	S	M	T	W	T	F	S

SEIZE THE DAY

MONDAY

TUESDAY

WEDNESDAY

THURSDAY

_____ / _____ / _____ TO _____ / _____ / _____

FRIDAY

SATURDAY

SUNDAY

TRIUMPHS OF THE WEEK

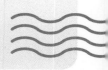

THIS WEEK

DON'T FORGET

QUESTIONS TO ASK

TO DO

CHART IT OUT

SYMPTOM, HABIT, OR MEDICINE

S	M	T	W	T	F	S

STRONGER THAN YESTERDAY

MONDAY

TUESDAY

WEDNESDAY

THURSDAY

_____ / _____ / _____ TO _____ / _____ / _____

FRIDAY

SATURDAY

SUNDAY

TRIUMPHS OF THE WEEK

THIS WEEK

DON'T FORGET

QUESTIONS TO ASK

TO DO

CHART IT OUT

SYMPTOM, HABIT, OR MEDICINE

S	M	T	W	T	F	S

ANYTHING IS POSSIBLE

MONDAY

TUESDAY

WEDNESDAY

THURSDAY

_____ / _____ / _____ TO _____ / _____ / _____

FRIDAY

SATURDAY

SUNDAY

TRIUMPHS OF THE WEEK

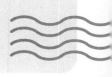

THIS WEEK

DON'T FORGET

QUESTIONS TO ASK

TO DO

CHART IT OUT

SYMPTOM, HABIT, OR MEDICINE

	S	M	T	W	T	F	S

I WILL RISE

- **MONDAY**

- **TUESDAY**

- **WEDNESDAY**

- **THURSDAY**

_____ / _____ / _____ TO _____ / _____ / _____

FRIDAY

SATURDAY

SUNDAY

TRIUMPHS OF THE WEEK

This planner was developed with cancer fighters, survivors, and caregivers who know just how tough the cancer fight can be.

YOU'VE GOT THIS!

Published by Sourcebooks
P.O. Box 4410, Naperville, Illinois 60567-4410
(630) 961-3900
sourcebooks.com

Printed and bound in China.
OGP 10 9 8 7 6 5 4 3 2 1

LET IT GO
LET IT GO
LET IT GO
LET IT GO
LET IT GO

STR⬤NG

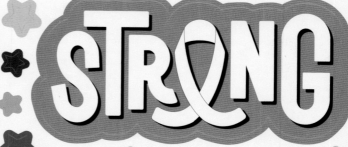

YES YOU CANCER

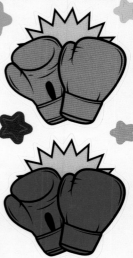

CANCER FIGHTER	CANCER FIGHTER	CANCER FIGHTER	CANCER FIGHTER	CANCER FIGHTER
CANCER FIGHTER	CANCER FIGHTER	CANCER FIGHTER	CANCER FIGHTER	CANCER FIGHTER
CANCER FIGHTER	CANCER FIGHTER	CANCER FIGHTER	CANCER FIGHTER	CANCER FIGHTER

NEVER GIVE UP

YOU GOT THIS

READY TO FIGHT. DETERMINED TO WIN.

RESET

BE BRAVE

RESET

BE BRAVE

RESET

DR. APPOINTMENT	DR. APPOINTMENT	DR. APPOINTMENT	REFRESH
DR. APPOINTMENT	DR. APPOINTMENT	DR. APPOINTMENT	BE BRAVE
DR. APPOINTMENT	DR. APPOINTMENT	DR. APPOINTMENT	REFRESH
DR. APPOINTMENT	DR. APPOINTMENT	DR. APPOINTMENT	BE BRAVE
DR. APPOINTMENT	DR. APPOINTMENT	DR. APPOINTMENT	REFRESH
DR. APPOINTMENT	DR. APPOINTMENT	DR. APPOINTMENT	BE BRAVE
DR. APPOINTMENT	DR. APPOINTMENT	DR. APPOINTMENT	
DR. APPOINTMENT	DR. APPOINTMENT	DR. APPOINTMENT	
DR. APPOINTMENT	DR. APPOINTMENT	DR. APPOINTMENT	
DR. APPOINTMENT	DR. APPOINTMENT	DR. APPOINTMENT	
DR. APPOINTMENT	DR. APPOINTMENT	DR. APPOINTMENT	
DR. APPOINTMENT	DR. APPOINTMENT	DR. APPOINTMENT	
DR. APPOINTMENT	DR. APPOINTMENT	DR. APPOINTMENT	
DR. APPOINTMENT	DR. APPOINTMENT	DR. APPOINTMENT	

DR. APPOINTMENT   DR. APPOINTMENT   DR. APPOINTMENT

DR. APPOINTMENT   DR. APPOINTMENT   DR. APPOINTMENT

DR. APPOINTMENT   DR. APPOINTMENT   DR. APPOINTMENT

DR. APPOINTMENT   DR. APPOINTMENT   DR. APPOINTMENT

DR. APPOINTMENT   DR. APPOINTMENT   DR. APPOINTMENT

DR. APPOINTMENT   DR. APPOINTMENT   DR. APPOINTMENT

DR. APPOINTMENT   DR. APPOINTMENT   DR. APPOINTMENT

DR. APPOINTMENT   DR. APPOINTMENT   DR. APPOINTMENT

DR. APPOINTMENT   DR. APPOINTMENT   DR. APPOINTMENT

DR. APPOINTMENT   DR. APPOINTMENT   DR. APPOINTMENT

DR. APPOINTMENT   DR. APPOINTMENT   DR. APPOINTMENT

DR. APPOINTMENT   DR. APPOINTMENT   DR. APPOINTMENT

DR. APPOINTMENT   DR. APPOINTMENT   DR. APPOINTMENT

DR. APPOINTMENT   DR. APPOINTMENT   DR. APPOINTMENT

SELF-CARE   START SMALL

SELF-CARE   START SMALL

SELF-CARE   START SMALL

SELF-CARE   START SMALL

SELF-CARE   START SMALL

SELF-CARE   START SMALL

SELF-CARE   START SMALL

SELF-CARE   START SMALL

IMPORTANT!	IMPORTANT!	IMPORTANT!	NOTE TO SELF	NOTE TO SELF
IMPORTANT!	IMPORTANT!	IMPORTANT!	NOTE TO SELF	NOTE TO SELF
IMPORTANT!	IMPORTANT!	IMPORTANT!	NOTE TO SELF	NOTE TO SELF
IMPORTANT!	IMPORTANT!	IMPORTANT!	NOTE TO SELF	NOTE TO SELF
IMPORTANT!	IMPORTANT!	IMPORTANT!	NOTE TO SELF	NOTE TO SELF
IMPORTANT!	IMPORTANT!	IMPORTANT!	NOTE TO SELF	NOTE TO SELF
IMPORTANT!	IMPORTANT!	IMPORTANT!	NOTE TO SELF	NOTE TO SELF
IMPORTANT!	IMPORTANT!	IMPORTANT!	NOTE TO SELF	NOTE TO SELF
IMPORTANT!	IMPORTANT!	IMPORTANT!	NOTE TO SELF	NOTE TO SELF
IMPORTANT!	IMPORTANT!	IMPORTANT!	NOTE TO SELF	NOTE TO SELF

YES YOU CAN **YES YOU CAN** **YES YOU CAN** **YES YOU CAN** **YES YOU CAN** **YES YOU CAN** **YES YOU CAN**

CELEBRATE	CELEBRATE	CELEBRATE	TREATMENT DAY	TREATMENT DAY
CELEBRATE	CELEBRATE	CELEBRATE	TREATMENT DAY	TREATMENT DAY
CELEBRATE	CELEBRATE	CELEBRATE	TREATMENT DAY	TREATMENT DAY
CELEBRATE	CELEBRATE	CELEBRATE	TREATMENT DAY	TREATMENT DAY
CELEBRATE	CELEBRATE	CELEBRATE	TREATMENT DAY	TREATMENT DAY
CELEBRATE	CELEBRATE	CELEBRATE	TREATMENT DAY	TREATMENT DAY
CELEBRATE	CELEBRATE	CELEBRATE	TREATMENT DAY	TREATMENT DAY
CELEBRATE	CELEBRATE	CELEBRATE	TREATMENT DAY	TREATMENT DAY
CELEBRATE	CELEBRATE	CELEBRATE	TREATMENT DAY	TREATMENT DAY
CELEBRATE	CELEBRATE	CELEBRATE	TREATMENT DAY	TREATMENT DAY

GRATEFUL	GRATEFUL
GRATEFUL	GRATEFUL
GRATEFUL	GRATEFUL
GRATEFUL	GRATEFUL
GRATEFUL	GRATEFUL
GRATEFUL	GRATEFUL
GRATEFUL	GRATEFUL

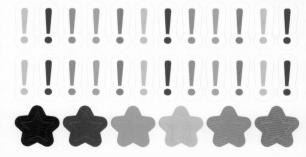

| TODAY IS A GOOD DAY | TODAY IS A GOOD DAY | TODAY IS A GOOD DAY | TODAY IS A GOOD DAY | TODAY IS A GOOD DAY | TODAY IS A GOOD DAY | TODAY IS A GOOD DAY |